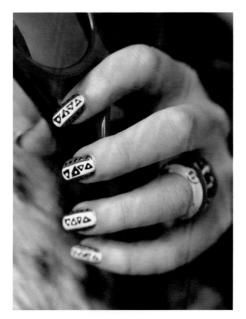

POLISH
YOU
PRETTY

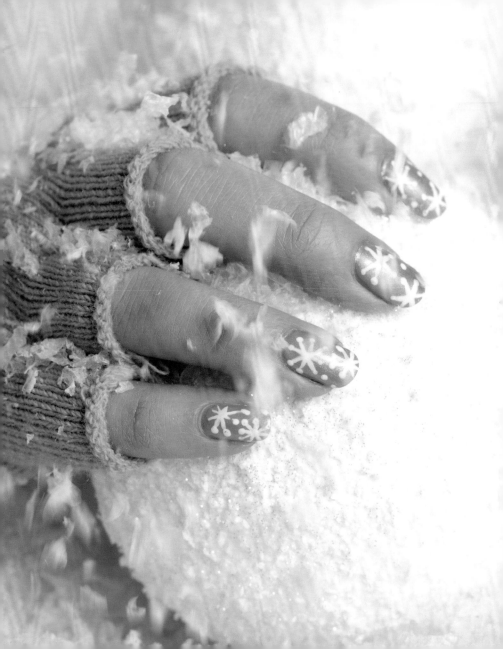

POLISH
YOU
PRETTY

24 stunning step-by-step nail art
designs you can create at home

Jenny Stencel & Danielle Black

With Photography by Terry Benson

LONDON • NEW YORK

Design Assistant Maria Lee-Warren
Editor Ellen Parnavelas
Production Manager Gordana Simakovic
Art Director Leslie Harrington
Editorial Director Julia Charles

Prop Stylist Rob Merrett
Nail Artist Maria Georgiou
Indexer Claire Hodgson

First published in 2013
by Ryland Peters & Small
20–21 Jockey's Fields
London WC1R 4BW
and
Ryland Peters & Small
519 Broadway, 5th Floor
New York, NY 10012

www.rylandpeters.com

10 9 8 7 6 5 4 3 2 1

ISBN: 978 1 84975 370 8

A CIP record for this book is available
from the British Library.

Library of Congress Cataloging-in-
Publication data has been applied for.

Printed in China.

About the Authors
Jenny Stencel and Danielle Black
have been friends since high school.
After bonding over their love of nail
polish and digital media, they started
their award-winning nail art blog
polishyoupretty.com – a blog that
features all the latest trends in nail art
and demonstrates the many fabulous
things you can do with nail polish.
Jenny and Danielle are both based
in Toronto, Canada.

CONTENTS

Tools & Techniques 6

Simple 18

Floral 44

Prints 62

Young at Heart 84

Seasonal 106

Resources & suppliers 124

Index 126

Acknowledgements 128

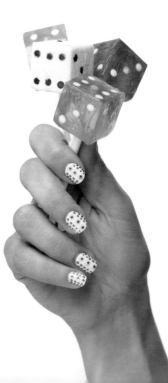

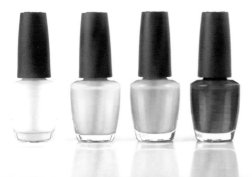

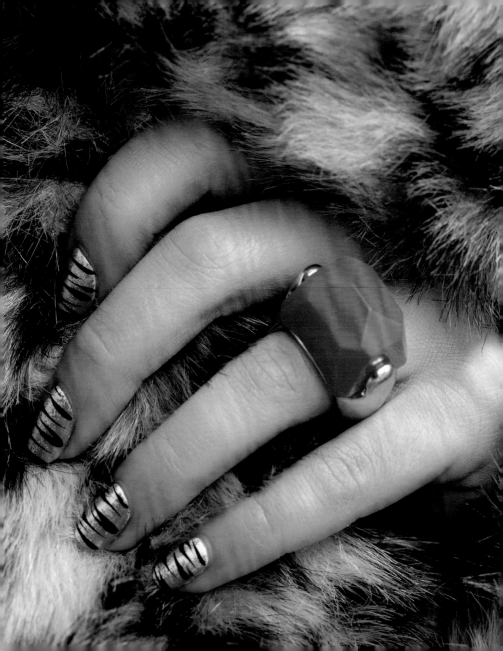

TOOLS & TECHNIQUES

WELCOME!

Welcome to the world of nail art! Nail art has become a growing trend over the last couple of years, and it has gone way beyond nail polish. Nail art is a fun and creative beauty trend that has grabbed the attention of everyone from fashion designers and bloggers to students and young professionals — everyone is doing it! And if you aren't doing nail art yourself, you at least have to admit that you've swooned over the latest designs and have wondered whether you could make your nails look that good too. Well we are here to show you that you can!

It's OK if you weren't the most talented student in your school art classes, and you don't have the steadiest of hands. You can still succeed in achieving all of these beautiful nail art designs. All you need is a little practice and the right tools. All the essentials you will need to get started are explained in this book. Polish You Pretty will have you looking and feeling like a nail art expert in no time. Enjoy!

POLISHES

If you don't already have an extensive nail polish collection don't worry! You can still achieve some great nail art designs with just a few simple colours. There are some essential shades that every polish collection should consist of – a neutral, a white and a black. These essentials will come in handy for a wide variety of different designs so start with these and build up your collection from here. When buying polishes, look for flat, creamy, opaque colours. And remember, there are often multiple steps to nail art designs, so you don't always need to paint two coats of each colour of polish – the more opaque the better the result.

Your base and top coat are two of the most important things when it comes to nail polish. These will keep your beautiful nail art designs looking lovely for days instead of hours. If you paint your nails often you should always use a base coat to keep you nails from staining. Base coats are meant to hold a polish to the nail – you should look for a base coat that is thin and dries fast. Your top coat should be a heavy-duty, fast-drying polish with a high shine. When applying these it's important to let your base coat dry before applying your colour polish, and to let your nail art set before applying a slick of top coat. Base and top coats will work differently for everyone, so it might take a while to find your perfect fit.

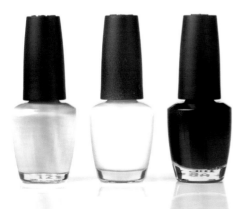

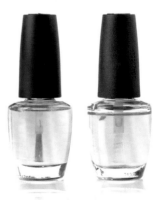

DOTTING TOOLS

A dotting tool is a good place to start when investing in nail art tools. Dotting tools are not essential for simple designs, but will still give professional results that will wow your friends. If you aren't yet confident enough in your nail art skills to purchase your own set of dotting tools, then using filed down cocktail sticks/toothpicks or the end of a hair pin works very well too. Once you do decide to purchase dotting tools, make sure you buy a range of sizes – small, medium and large.

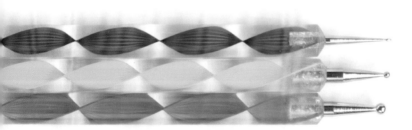

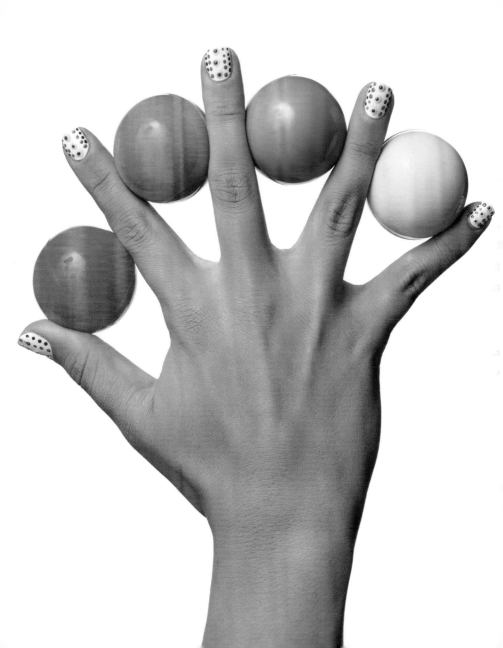

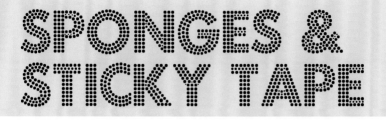

SPONGES & STICKY TAPE

We love sponging on our nails! It's very easy and delivers impressive results. When sponging your nails you can simply purchase make-up sponges (of the type used to apply foundation to your face) and cut them into smaller pieces. When cutting your sponges, make sure you cut them in a size that will cover the width of your nail to achieve full coverage.

Sticky tape will come in handy many times in this book. For beginners, using tape to perfect your lines will be a good alternative to free-hand drawing. If a design is extra messy, then using tape to cover the skin around your nails will save you some time and effort at the end when it comes to cleaning up.

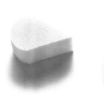
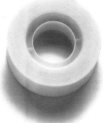

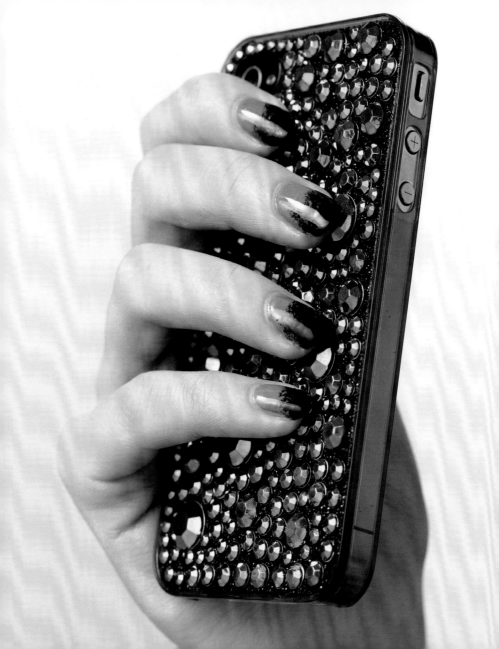

NAIL ART BRUSHES

Nail art brushes are not only used for more difficult nail art designs, but for simple ones as well. Investing in one or multiple brushes is a good idea if you want to be able to paint a variety of different designs. If you are going to purchase a set of nail art brushes, make sure to get two or three different sizes because some nail art designs call for tiny details, where others simply need a basic outline. If you don't have a steady hand and aren't sure if you want to invest in nail art brushes, then purchasing a nail art pen in a basic colour is the best way to learn and refine the necessary skills to paint freehand with a brush.

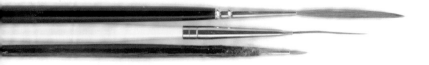

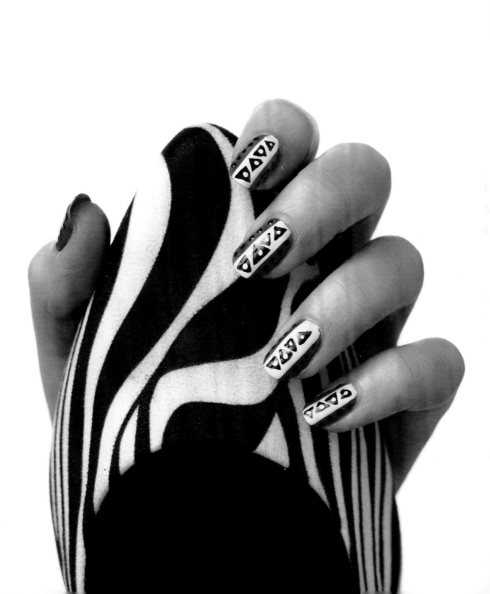

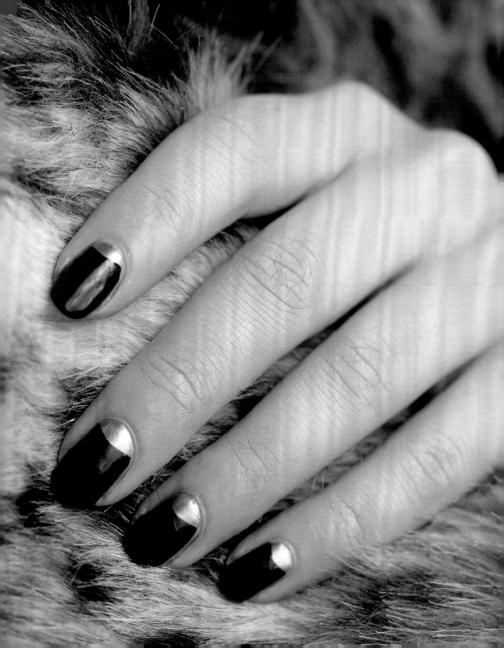

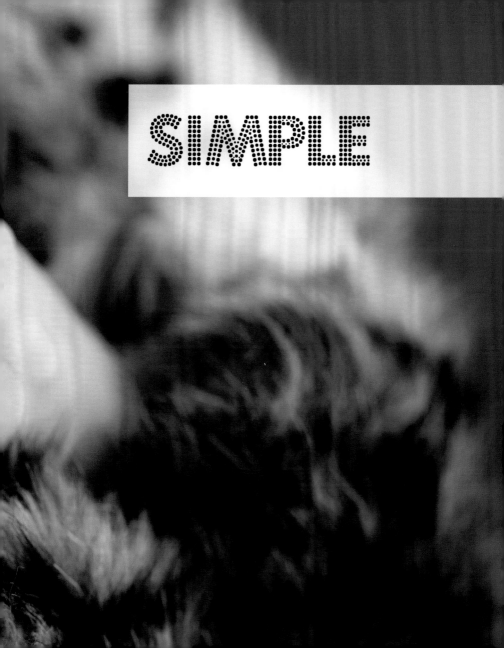

SIMPLE

LOVE nail art, but don't know where to start? This chapter will guide you through some of our most simple designs to help you learn the basic skills you need to create fabulous nail art – and we promise, simple does NOT have to mean boring!

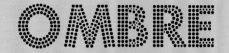

OMBRE

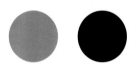

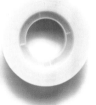

YOU WILL NEED

- Top and base coats
- Sponge
- Sticky tape

COLOURS

- Neutral
- Black

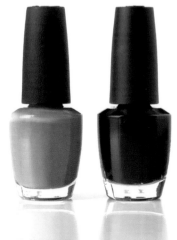

This design is high in the **FASHION** stakes! It only takes a few minutes to achieve so you can have nails worthy of a Paris runway in the time it takes to sip a glass of Champagne backstage!

1 Apply a base coat and when dry, paint your nails with two coats of the neutral polish using the brush from the bottle. Once dry, put tape around all of your nails – this will allow for an easy clean-up.

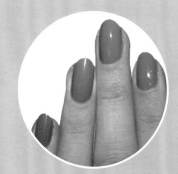

2 Cut a make-up sponge into thin slices. Dip the sponge into the black nail polish, then dab the sponge on a piece of scrap paper to remove excess polish.

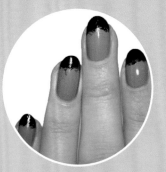

3 Dab your sponge onto the tip of each nail, starting with a heavier pressure and getting lighter as you get closer to the base. Repeat with all of your nails, making sure all the tips are solid black. Once you have finished all your nails and they have completely dried, remove the tape and apply a top coat.

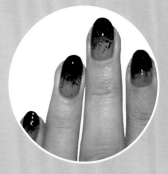

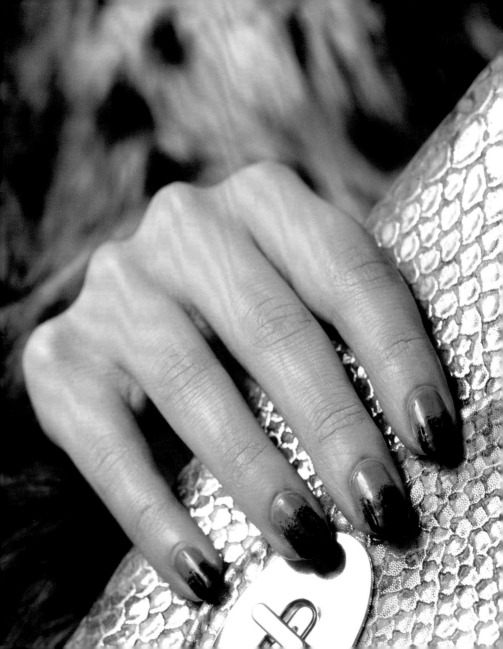

POLKA DOT POWER

YOU WILL NEED

- Top and base coats
- Dotting tools shown

COLOURS

- White
- Yellow
- Blue
- Red

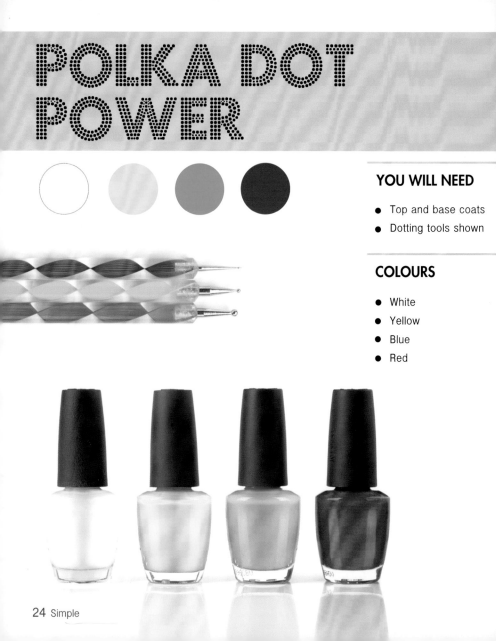

Ready to roll some **DICE**! Take a gamble on this design and add a playful touch to your manicure. You can experiment with different colour combinations but opaque white is always a great colour to use as a background.

1 Apply a base coat and when dry, paint your nails with two coats of the white polish, using the brush from the bottle. Allow to dry completely.

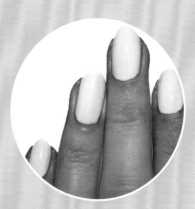

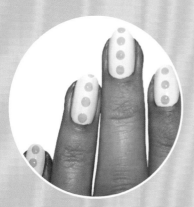

2 Using a large dotting tool dipped in the yellow polish, dot four large polka dots down the middle of each nail.

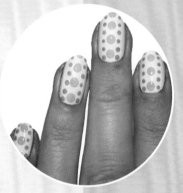

3 Using a medium dotting tool, dipped in the blue polish, dot six medium polka dots on either side of the row of yellow dots on each nail.

4 Using a small dotting tool, dipped in the red polish, dot a row of tiny red dots on both outer edges of each of your nails. Finish the design by placing a tiny red dot in the middle of each large yellow one and allow to dry. Once all the dots have completely dried, seal the design with top coat.

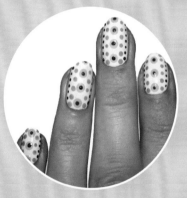

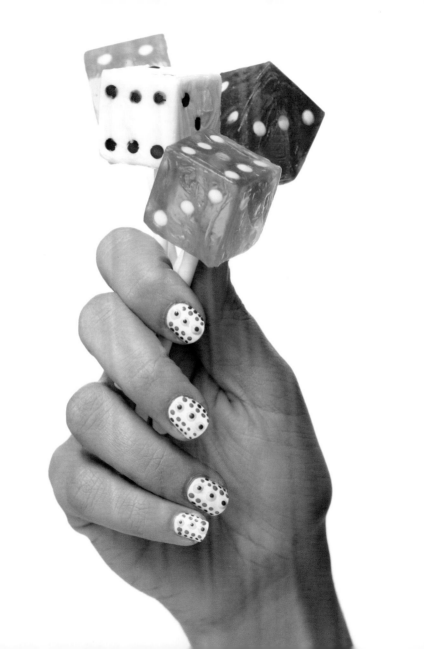

SPLATTER

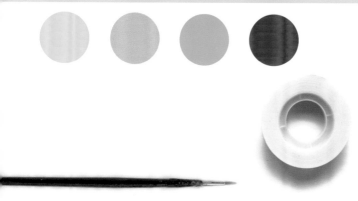

YOU WILL NEED

- Top and base coats
- Nail art brush shown
- Sticky tape

COLOURS

- Yellow
- Neutral
- Metallic blue
- Orange

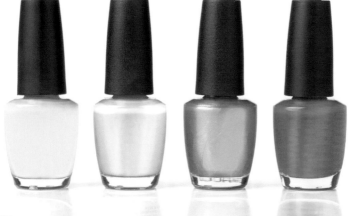

Learn to thrive in the **CHAOS**! This design is one of the most fun to do because the messier you are, the better your end result will be. If you feel nervous about the more intricate designs – we recommend you throw yourself into this one!

1 Make sure to put down some newspaper before you work – you'll thank us later! Apply a base coat and when dry, paint your nails with two coats of the neutral polish. Allow to dry completely and then put tape around all of your nails to allow for an easy clean up – things are about to get extremely messy!

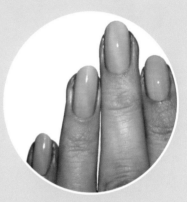

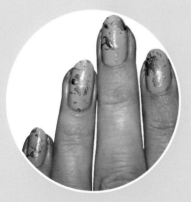

2 Using a nail art brush dipped into the blue polish, flick the brush over your nails so that the blue polish splatters over them. Make sure you have a generous amount of polish on your brush. Repeat until there are blue splatters on all of your nails. Allow to dry completely. Clean the brush with nail polish remover.

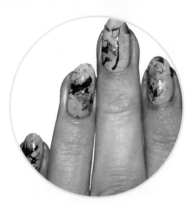

3 Repeat the previous step using the yellow polish and allow to dry. Clean the brush with nail polish remover before repeating with the orange polish. With the addition of each new colour, try to strategically flick the polish to create splatters in the uncovered areas so that your nails are covered evenly with a colourful pattern. Allow to dry completely. Remove the tape and clean up any excess polish on your fingers. A pointed cottonbud/Q-tip works well. Seal with top coat.

WREAK SOME HAVOC!

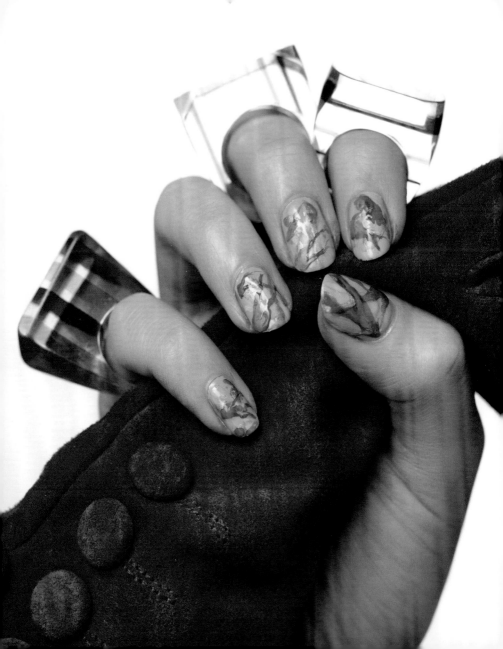

HALF MOON

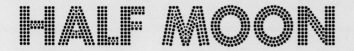

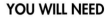

YOU WILL NEED

- Top and base coats
- Nail art brush shown

COLOURS

- Metallic silver
- Dark red

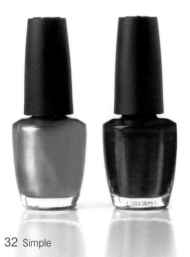

This design is pure **THEATRE** so don't be afraid to take centre stage on your next night out. Flash these fabulous fingertips and get ready to take your curtain call!

1 Apply a base coat and when dry, paint your nails with one coat of the metallic silver polish. Allow to dry completely.

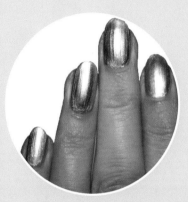

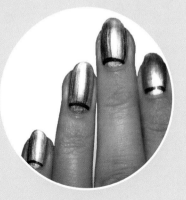

2 Using a nail art brush dipped in the dark red polish, paint a 'U' shape around the base of each of your nails. Using the brush from the polish bottle, fill in the rest of all your nails with the dark red, leaving the silver half-moons at the base of each nail.

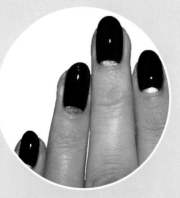

3 Allow your nails to dry completely, then seal with a top coat.

Tip: If you don't have a steady hand you can try using sticky tape to create an outline of your half moon in step 2, just make sure your design has dried before removing the tape. This will leave you with a nice clean line.

ALWAYS MAKE A DRAMATIC ENTRANCE

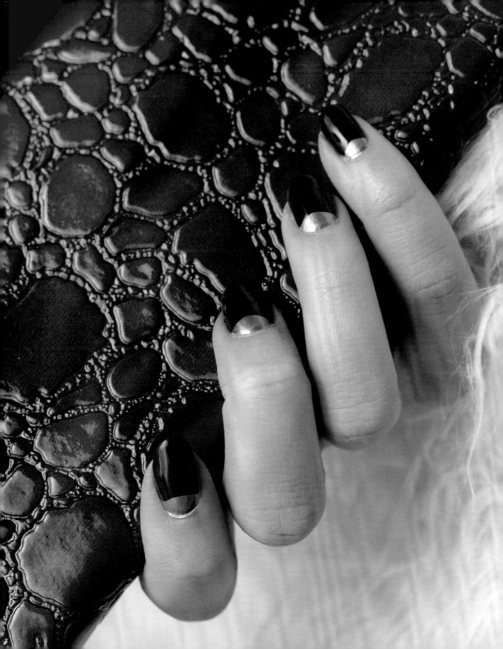

STAINED GLASS

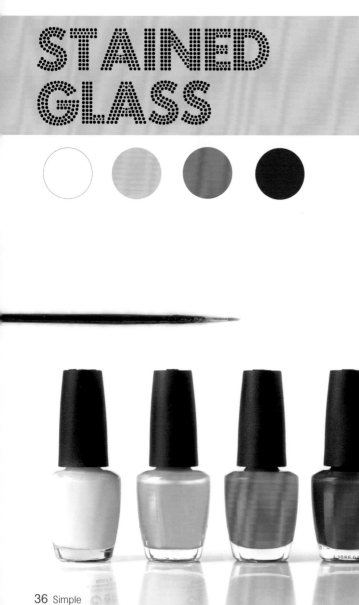

YOU WILL NEED

- Top and base coats
- Nail art brush shown

COLOURS

- White
- Pale pink
- Medium pink
- Dark pink

Are you a nail art amateur? You'll soon see the light once you've tried this simple yet **ILLUMINATING** design. It's perfect for all levels of ability as it hides the imperfections at the end!

1 After applying a base coat, paint the bottom half of each of your nails with a different shade of pink, alternating colours from nail to nail. If you are new to nail art it is best to paint your nails from lightest to darkest. Allow to dry.

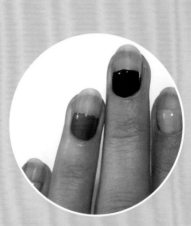

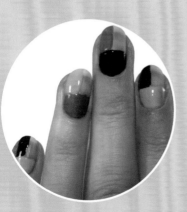

2 Paint the top left-hand quarter of each of your nails with a different shade of pink to the base. You can paint free-hand using the brush from the bottle or use a nail art brush to ensure cleaner lines. The lines do not have to be perfect, as you can use the final step to clean things up. Allow to dry.

LET
THERE BE
BRIGHT!

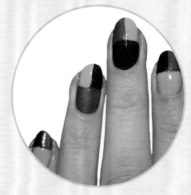

3 Repeat step 2 with the top right-hand quarters of your nails, using a contrasting shade of pink.

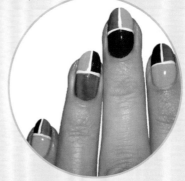

4 Allow your nails to dry completely. Dip your nail art brush in your white polish and draw a horizontal, then a vertical line to outline each of the panels of pink on all of your nails. Allow your nails to dry, then seal with a heavy-duty top coat.

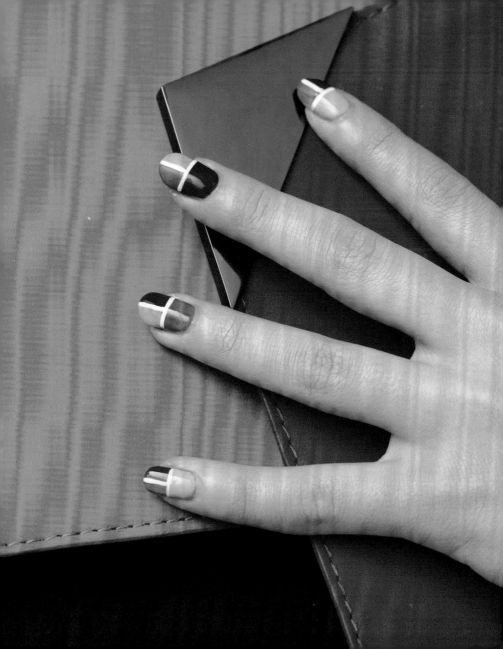

MAGIC MIXING

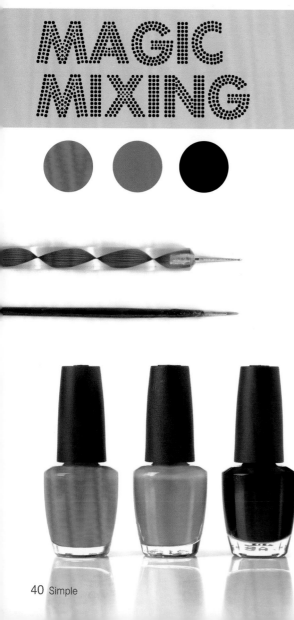

YOU WILL NEED

- Top and base coats
- Dotting tool shown
- Nail art brush shown

COLOURS

- Pink
- Purple
- Black

Want to see a **TRICK**? Get ready to take your nail art to the next level by combining two tantalizing techniques in one design. Combining stripes and dots is easier than it looks, and the results are guaranteed to amaze your friends!

1 Apply a base coat and when dry, paint your nails with two coats of the purple polish using the brush from the bottle. Allow to dry. Take the pink polish and, again using the brush from the bottle, paint the left side of your nails to provide a contrast to the purple.

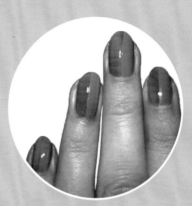

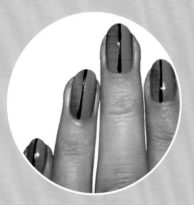

2 Using a nail art brush dipped into the black polish, paint a fine black outline between the pink and purple panels. Allow to dry.

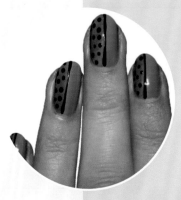

3 Dip the dotting tool into the black polish and dot the pink side of your nails with spaced polka dots. Make sure your dots aren't too close together and that you can still see the pink polish. Allow to dry.

4 Using the nail art brush dipped in the black polish, paint five diagonal lines over the purple panel on each of your nails. Allow to dry completely, then seal with top coat. Tada!

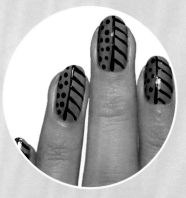

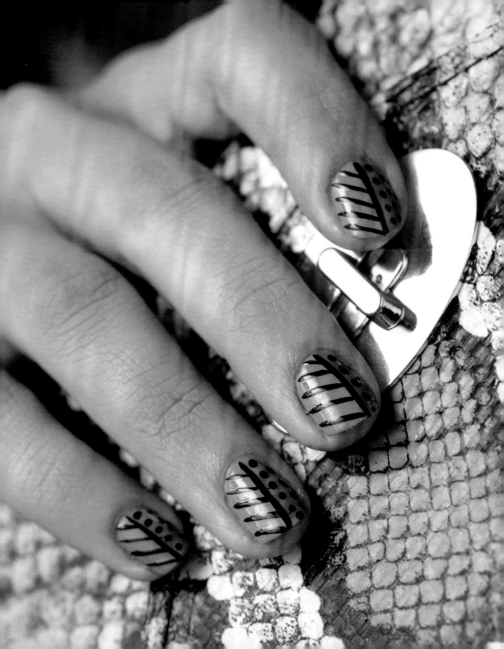

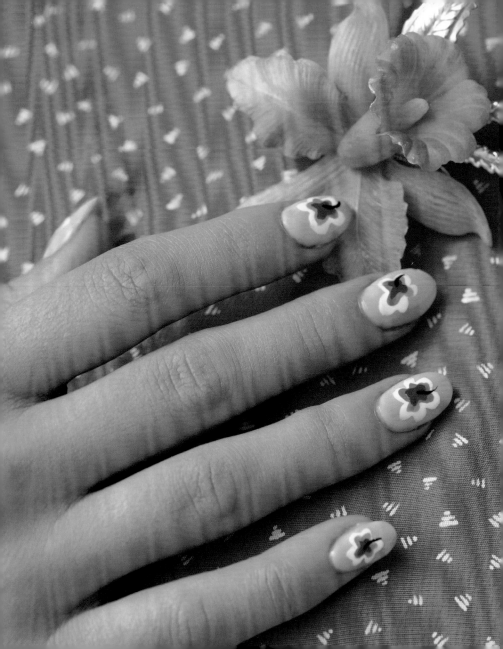

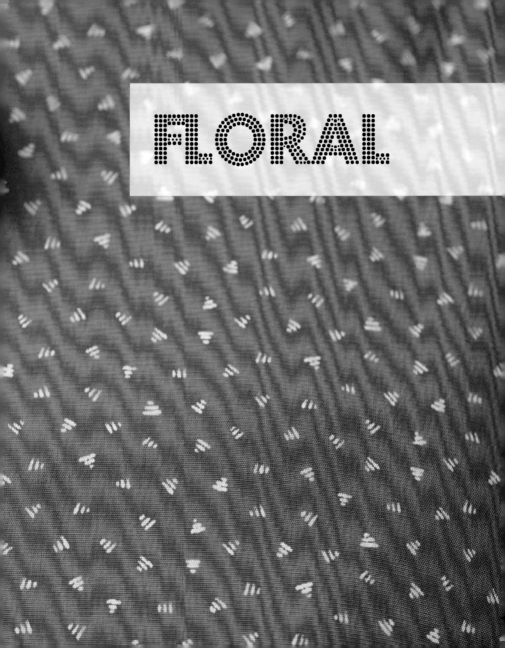

FLORAL

FLORAL

Prepare to have this book permanently open on this chapter during the spring and summer months. Floral nail art designs will brighten up your fingertips and are designs that really let you get creative with an explosion of colour. Florals require a lot of free-hand work, so be sure to have your nail art brush to hand and get ready to BLOOM.

SMELL THE ROSES

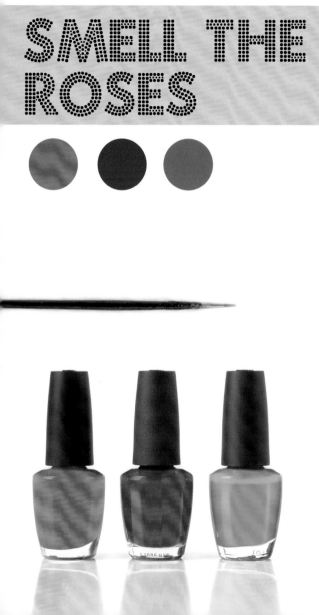

YOU WILL NEED

- Top and base coats
- Nail art brush shown

COLOURS

- Light pink
- Dark pink
- Green

Create your very own rose garden in full bloom with this timelessly **ELEGANT** floral design. If you really want to come up smelling of roses, try using a scented top coat!

1 Apply a base coat and when dry, paint your nails with two coats of the light pink polish.

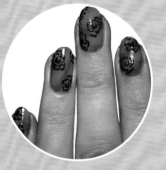

2 Once the base colour has dried you can begin with the flower design. Dip a nail art brush in the dark pink polish, and paint two or three small 'C' shapes on each of your nails where you'd like the middle of each rose to be. With the 'C' shape at the centre, paint four crescent shapes all the way around each 'C' shape to create the petals. Add one or two more petals on the outside of the crescents to add more volume to your roses. Allow to dry.

3 Using the green polish, paint small leaves around the roses in the spaces surrounding the flowers. Allow your nails to dry completely, then seal with top coat.

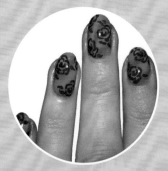

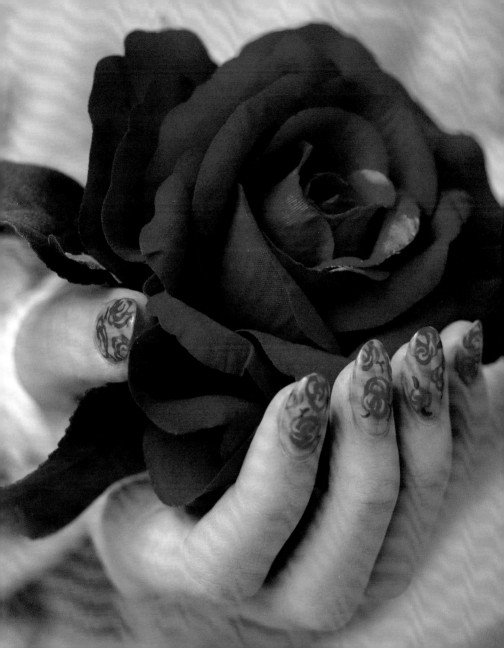

ROSEBUDS

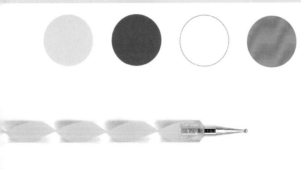

YOU WILL NEED

- Top and base coats
- Dotting tool shown
- Nail art brush shown

COLOURS

- Mint green
- Dark green
- White
- Pink

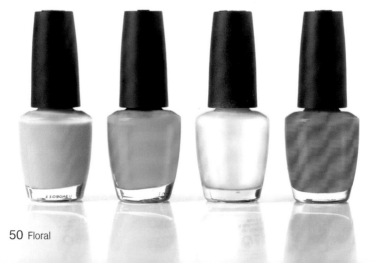

This **VINTAGE** design is pretty-as-a-picture. Use soft pastel shades to create a delicate and feminine look, perfect for an afternoon tea party. One lump or two?

1 Apply a base coat and allow to dry. Paint your nails with one or two coats of the light polish and allow to dry completely.

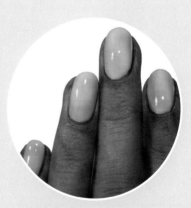

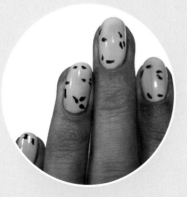

2 Once your base colour has dried, dip the nail art brush in the dark green polish. Paint a few small, irregular shapes all over each of your nails to create the leaves for your roses.

3 Dip the dotting tool in the white polish and dot a large white dot in the middle of one or two groups of dark green leaves on each of your nails. Allow to dry completely.

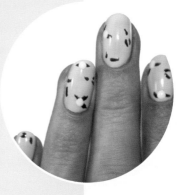

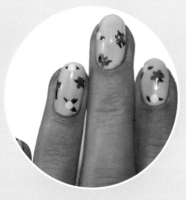

4 Clean the nail art brush with nail polish remover, then use the brush to paint one or two small, pink flowers in the middle of the remaining groups of dark green leaves on each of your nails. Allow to dry completely.

5 Dip the dotting tool in the dark pink polish and put a medium-sized dot in the middle of each of the large, white dots. Allow your nails to dry completely, then seal with a top coat.

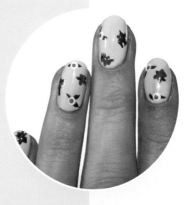

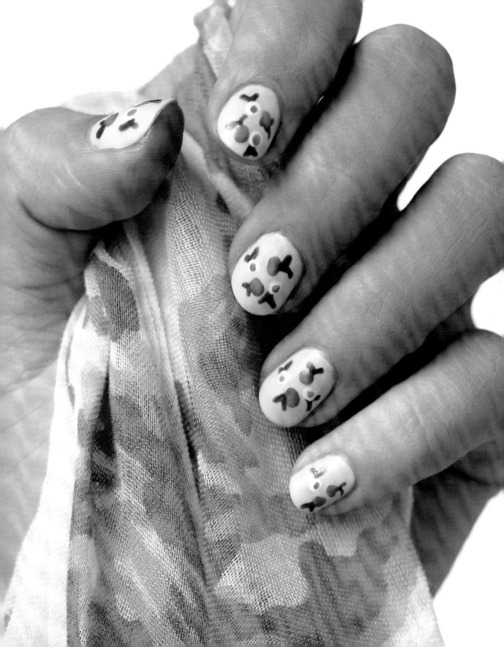

ALOHA

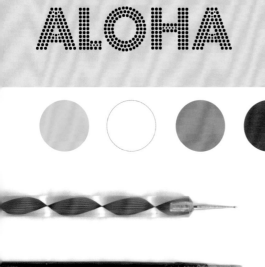

YOU WILL NEED

- Top and base coats
- Dotting tool shown
- Nail art brush shown

COLOURS

- Yellow
- White
- Light and dark pink
- Black

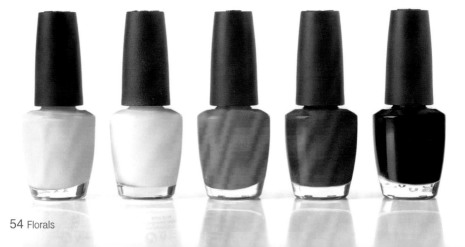

Who needs to go to a Hawaiian **LUAU** when you can bring the poolside party to your manicure? The only rule for this fun, fun, fun design is the brighter the better!

1 Apply a base coat and once dry, paint your nails with two coats of the yellow polish. Allow to dry completely.

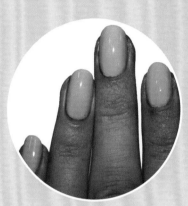

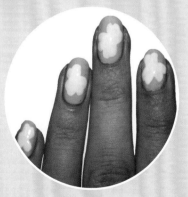

2 Take the white polish and using the brush from the bottle, create the white outer petals of the flower. Create three long, wide shapes with heart-shaped tops, bringing all the brush strokes into the middle of the design. Allow to dry completely.

3 Dip the nail art brush in the light pink polish and paint a starburst shape in the centre of each of the white flowers. Allow to dry.

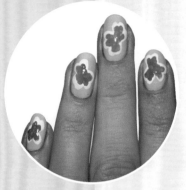

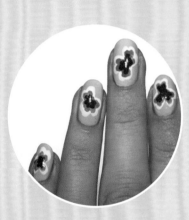

4 Clean the nail art brush with nail polish remover and paint a smaller, starburst shape in the middle of each flower using the darker pink polish. Allow to dry.

5 Clean the nail art brush with nail polish remover. Dip it in the black polish and paint a thin line coming from the middle of the tropical flower on each of your nails. Allow to dry completely and seal with top coat!

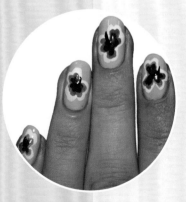

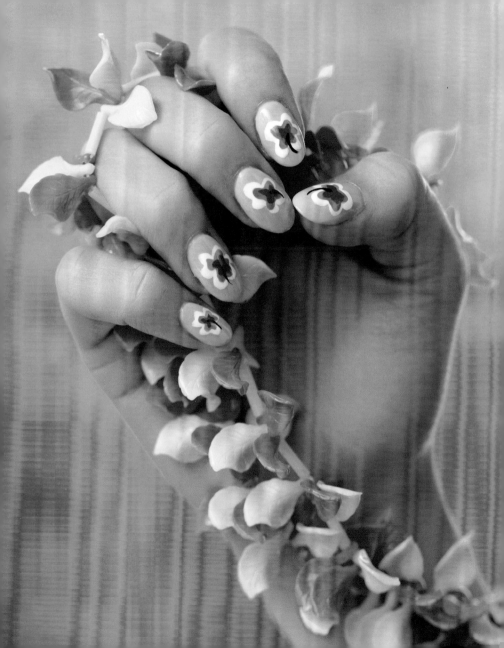

PRETTY PEONIES

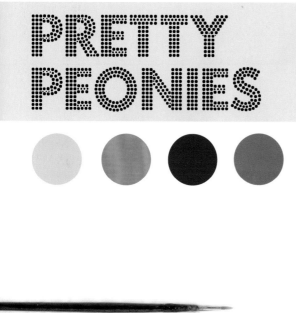

YOU WILL NEED

- Top and base coats
- Nail art brush shown

COLOURS

- Light green
- Bright pink
- Dark pink
- Dark green

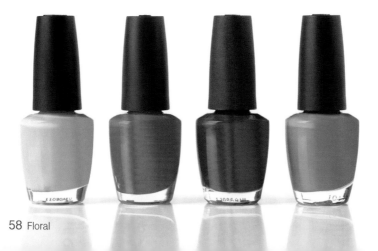

Paint a prize-winning floral display of peony **PETALS** and prove to your friends that you are truly green-fingered. Fresh, floral and fabulous – this design screams summer!

1 Apply a base coat and when dry, paint your nails with two coats of the light green polish. (A teal based polish works best for this and will really let your pink and red colours sing.)

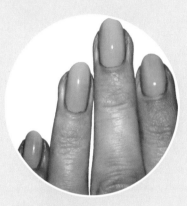

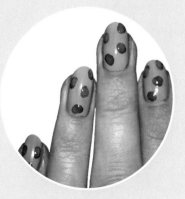

2 Dip the nail art brush into the pink polish and paint four large dots on each of your nails. Allow to dry completely. Clean the nail art brush with nail polish remover.

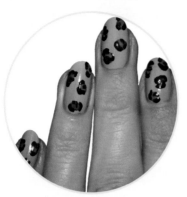

3 Dip the nail art brush in the red polish and paint small semi-circles around three sides of the dots, dragging one line into the middle of each dot. Allow to dry completely.

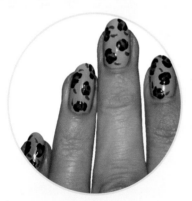

4 Dip the nail art brush into the dark green polish and paint small leaves around the peonies (in the spaces surrounding the flowers). Allow to dry completely and seal with top coat.

SUMMER IN FULL BLOOM!

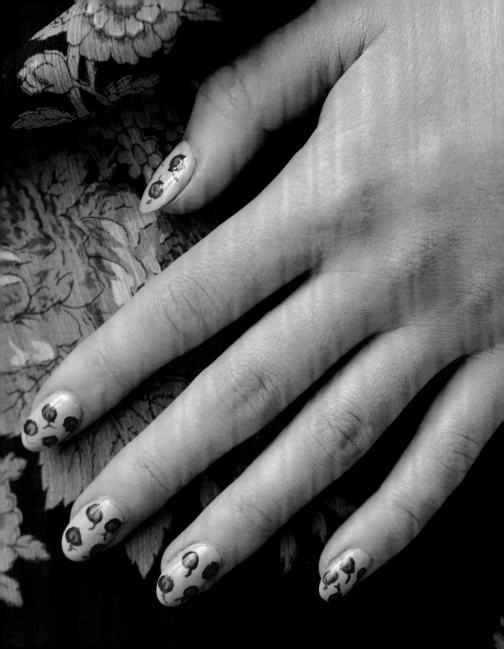

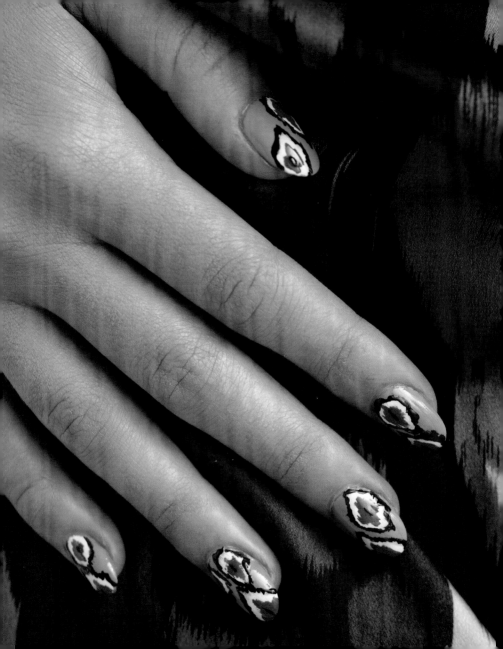

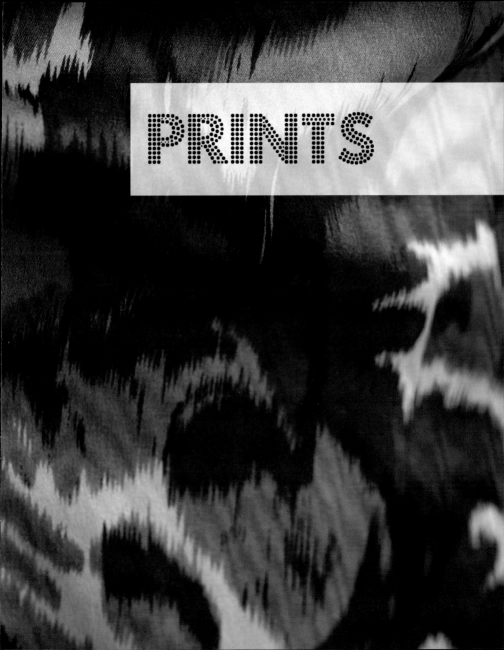

PRINTS

PRINTS

Replicating a fashion print is hugely popular in nail art. Here we've outlined some favourites that will have you well on your way to becoming a nail art EXPERT. You don't have to use classic colours to make these designs work. It's time to break out your BRIGHTEST shades and have some fun!

TIGER BRIGHT

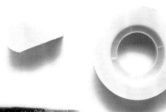

YOU WILL NEED

- Top and base coats
- Nail art brush shown
- Sponge
- Sticky tape

COLOURS

- White
- Orange
- Black

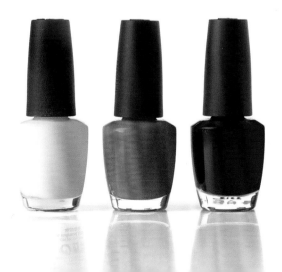

It's time to bring out your inner beast. You'll be more than ready for a rumble in the urban **JUNGLE** with this tiger-bright nail design. Bang on trend and fun yet sophisticated – get ready to roar!

1 Apply a base coat and once dry, paint all your nails with two coats of the white polish. Allow to dry. Protect your cuticles with sticky tape.

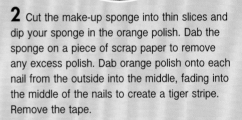

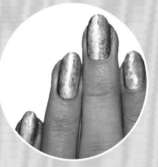

2 Cut the make-up sponge into thin slices and dip your sponge in the orange polish. Dab the sponge on a piece of scrap paper to remove any excess polish. Dab orange polish onto each nail from the outside into the middle, fading into the middle of the nails to create a tiger stripe. Remove the tape.

3 Dip a nail art brush into the black polish and paint on black tiger stripes. Remember to lighten the brush stroke near the end of each stripe to create a point. Also, to vary the design, try adding a few 'V'-shaped stripes as well. Allow to dry completely and seal with top coat. Get ready to roar!

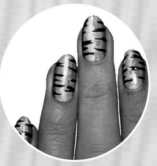

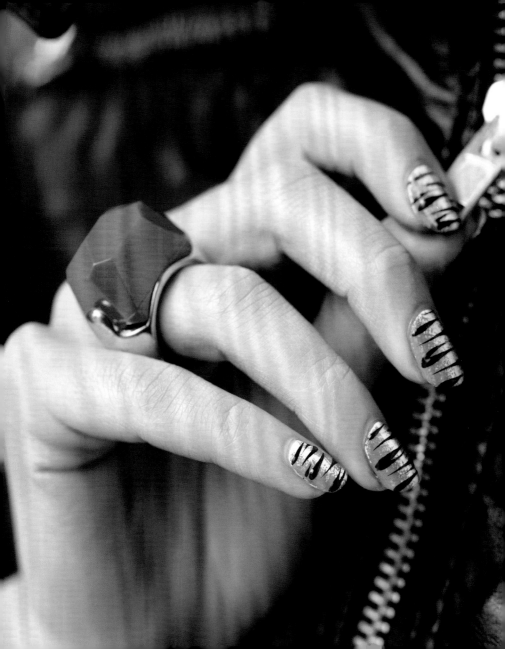

LEAPIN' LEOPARD

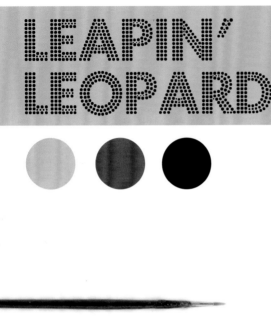

YOU WILL NEED

- Top and base coats
- Nail art brush shown

COLOURS

- Tan or beige
- Red
- Black

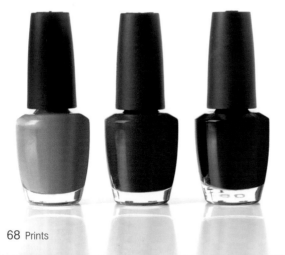

This timeless **ANIMAL** pattern never goes out of vogue. Go with the classic colours we've used here or make your own fashion statement with a pallete of shocking pinks or electric blues.

1 Apply a base coat and let dry. Paint your nails with two coats of the tan or beige polish.

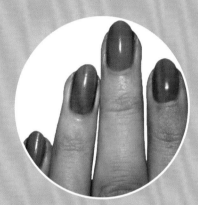

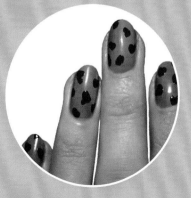

2 Once the base colour has dried, use a nail brush dipped in the red polish to create dots or smudges on each nail. The shapes do not have to be uniform, as different shapes will make the finish more interesting.

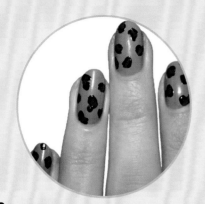

3 Using a nail art brush dipped in the black polish, draw a partial outline around all the red spots. Vary the shape of this outline, drawing either a 'C' or an 'L', picking up the brush as you work.

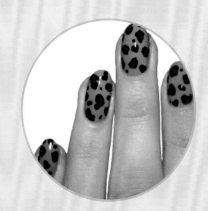

4 Finish by adding some black polka dots or smudges — you can use a filed down toothpick/cocktail stick to do this — inbetween the print. Allow to dry and seal with top coat.

IT'S TIME TO FOLLOW YOUR ANIMAL INSTINCTS!

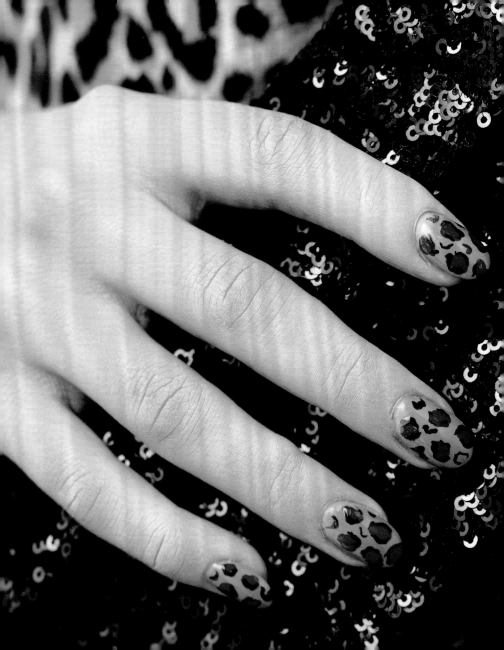

IKAT

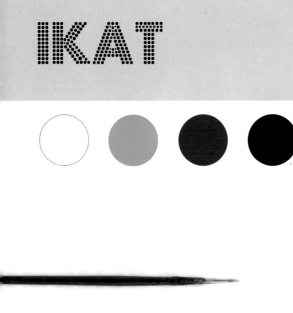

YOU WILL NEED

- Top and base coats
- Nail art brush shown

COLOURS

- White
- Blue
- Red
- Black

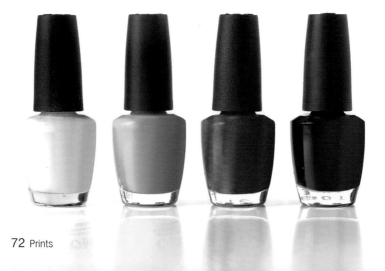

Lovers of interior **DESIGN** rejoice! This beautiful ikat print is the perfect accessory to any outfit. The technique is easy and leaves plenty of room for error, so if you are a novice be sure to give this one a try!

1 Apply a base coat and when dry, paint your nails with two coats of the blue polish. Allow to dry completely.

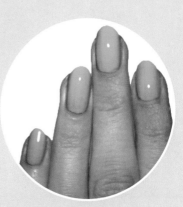

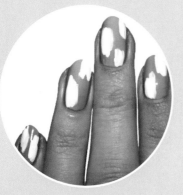

2 Once your base colour has dried, dip the nail art brush in the white polish and draw shapes on your nails as shown here – two or three long and narrow shapes will work best. Clean the nail brush with nail polish remover.

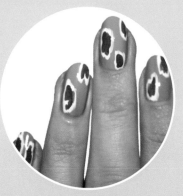

3 Dip the nail brush into the red polish and fill in the centres of the white spaces with a jagged shape, leaving a border around the outside. You don't have to be precise with this step, any shape will do. Clean the brush with nail polish remover.

4 Next, dip the nail art brush in the black polish and paint long straight strokes around the design, all pointing vertically. Paint all the way around the white shapes to create borders. To finish, paint a black small stroke in the middle of each one. Allow to dry completely and seal with top coat.

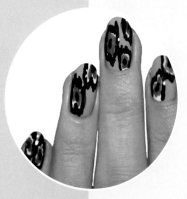

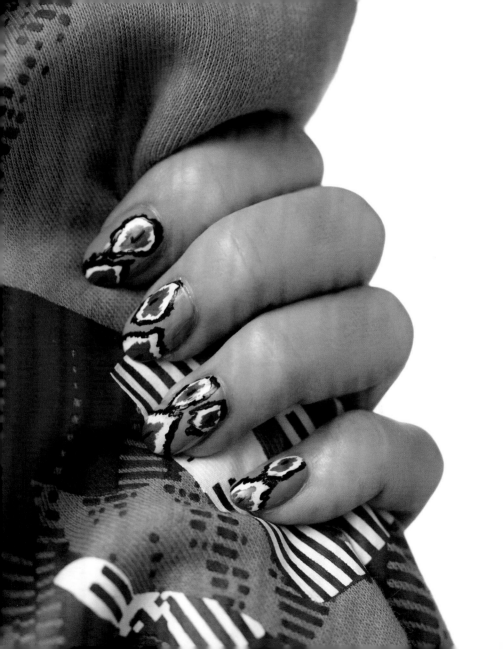

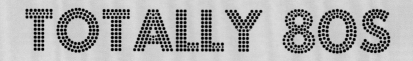
TOTALLY 80S

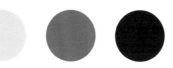

YOU WILL NEED

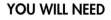

- Top and base coats
- Nail art brush shown

COLOURS

- Light green
- Mauve
- Bright pink

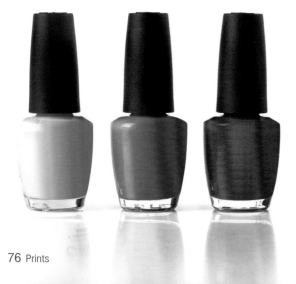

Here is a design for when you want to channel your inner 80s **DISCO** diva. Anything goes here colourwise – try neon polishes for a bang on-trend look or use a silver glitter top coat to create some mirror-ball brilliance!

1 Apply a base coat and allow it to dry. Take the light green polish and using the brush from the bottle, paint one third of each nail as shown. This line does not have to be perfect.

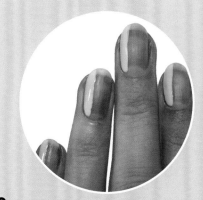

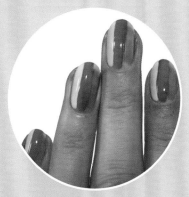

2 Take the mauve polish and using the brush from the bottle, paint a stripe down the centre of each nail. Dab a little extra of the mauve on the border of where the two polishes meet.

2 Take the pink polish and using the brush from the bottle, paint a third and final stripe as shown. Dab a little extra of the pink on the border of where the two polishes meet.

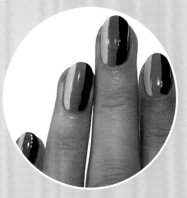

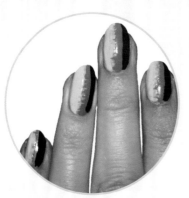

3 Using a nail art brush, drag the mauve into the green to create a jagged edge effect.

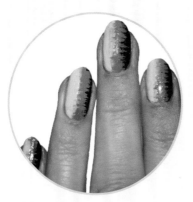

4 Repeat by dragging the pink polish into the mauve. Allow to dry completely and seal with top coat or finish with a slick of glitter-flecked clear polish for some disco dazzle!

LIKE, IT'S SO TOTALLY 80s! WHATEVER!

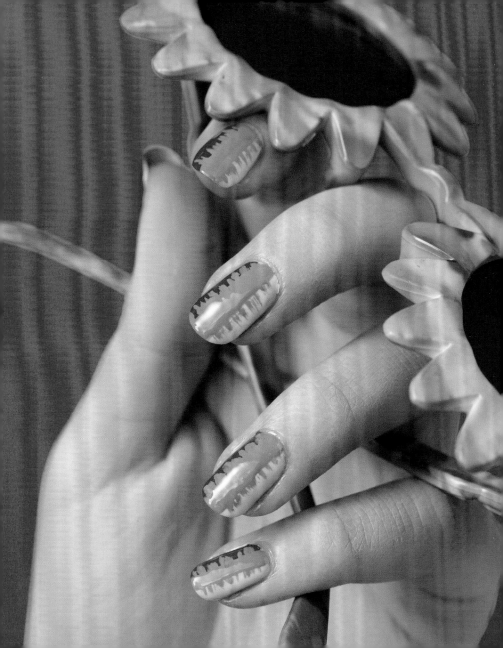

TRIBAL

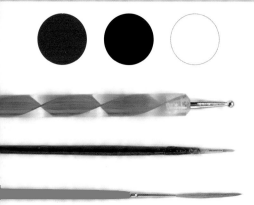

YOU WILL NEED

- Top and base coats
- Dotting tool shown
- Nail art brushes shown

COLOURS

- Bright pink
- Black
- White

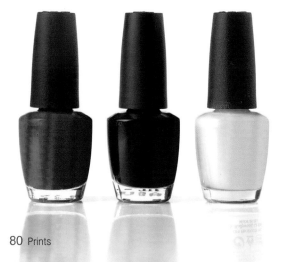

Tribal-inspired patterns are big news on the runway and in nail art just now so you'll **DRUM** up plenty of admiration from your fashionista friends with this eye-catching design.

1 Apply a base coat and when dry paint your nails with two coats of the bright red polish. Allow to dry completely.

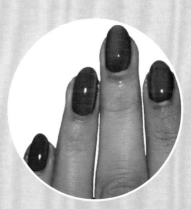

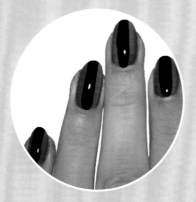

2 Take the black polish and use a regular nail art brush to paint a wide stripe down the centre of each of your nails.

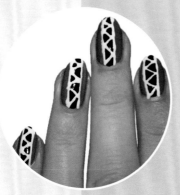

3 Dip the fine nail art brush in the white polish and paint over the black stripe of polish, leaving small black triangles peaking through. Don't worry too much about making these perfect.

4 To finish, use a dotting tool dipped in white polish to add a small dot to the centre of each black triangle. Clean the tool and dip it into the black polish. Add small dots along the length of the red stripes. Allow to dry completely and seal with top coat.

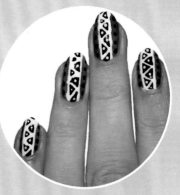

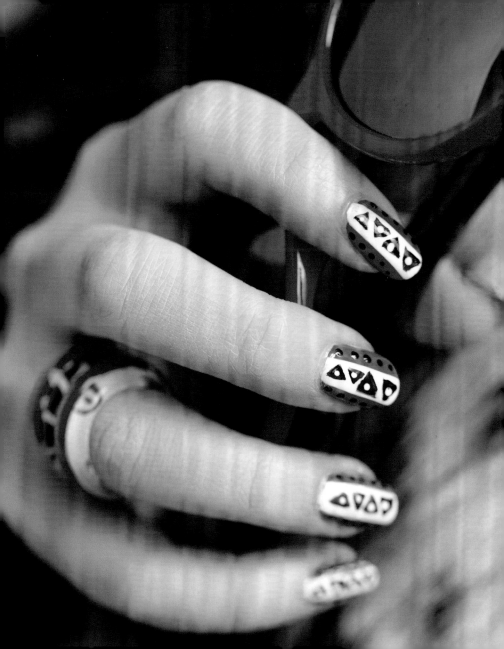

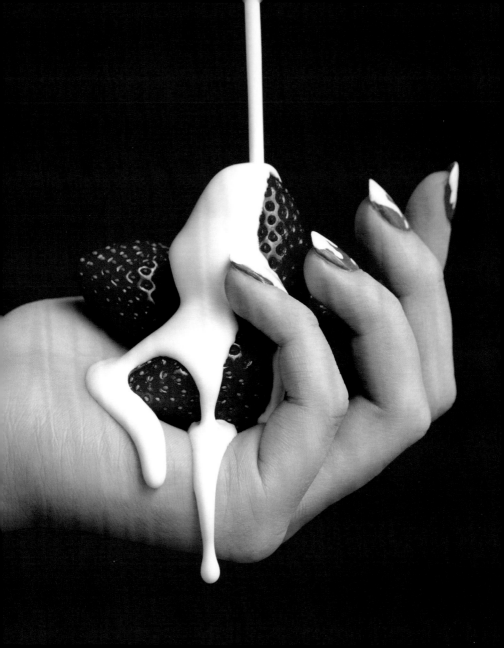

YOUNG AT HEART

YOUNG AT HEART

We both find that painting our nails takes us back to our CHILDHOOD. We used to break into our mom's make-up bags and steal their brightest polish colours all the time. Our nails didn't end up looking the best of course, but we wish we could've worn a few of these FUN designs growing up. We're all really still kids at heart, aren't we?

MELTING

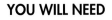

YOU WILL NEED

- Top and base coats
- Nail art brush shown

COLOURS

- Bright red
- Opaque white

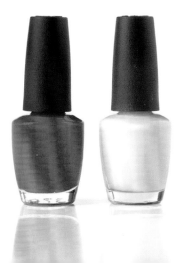

Everyone remembers ordering their favourite **ICE CREAM** as a kid and having it melt and drip down their hands before they had a chance to eat it all. This nostalgic design will bring back plenty of sweet soda fountain memories.

1 Apply a base coat and when dry, paint your nails with two coats of the red polish using the brush from the bottle. (We chose this candy bright red, but a fondant pink or chocolate brown works just as well.)

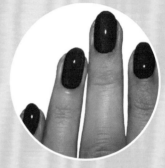

2 Wait until the red polish has completely dried before adding the drips. To do this, take the white polish and, using a nail art brush, paint on the outline shape. Using the brush from the polish bottle, fill in the rest with thick, even strokes. Drop a few extra tiny drips on the nail to finish the effect.

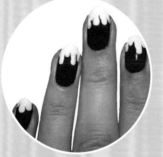

3 Once the drips are completely dry, seal your nail design with a layer of high-shine top coat and you're done! Sugary, sweet and good enough to eat!

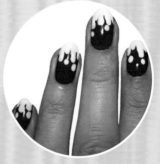

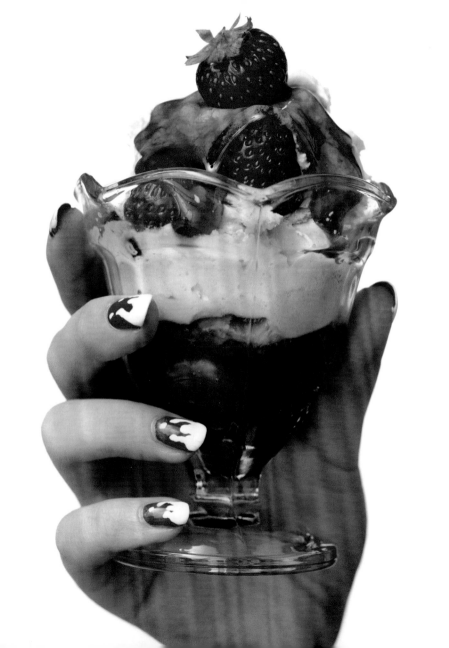

STRAWBERRY FIELDS

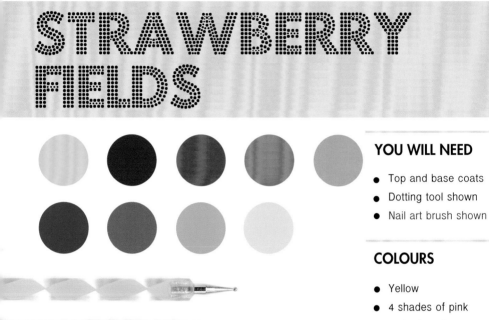

YOU WILL NEED

- Top and base coats
- Dotting tool shown
- Nail art brush shown

COLOURS

- Yellow
- 4 shades of pink
- 4 shades of green

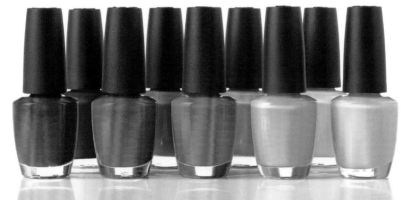

We all love juicy summer **STRAWBERRIES** so why not paint a punnet on your fingertips so that you can enjoy them all year round? This fresh and fruity design reminds us of heading to the strawberry fields to pick our own as kids!

1 Apply a base coat and when dry, paint each nail with two coats of a different shade using the brush from the bottle. Graduate from the pale pink through to the dark red. (You can paint your thumb to match your pinkie!)

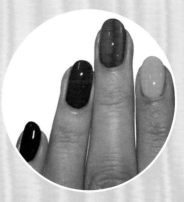

2 To add the strawberry seed effect, take the yellow polish, and using a small dotting tool, add polka dots all over each nail (we find that spacing them like a '5' on a dice tends to be the best way to space them evenly). Allow to dry completely.

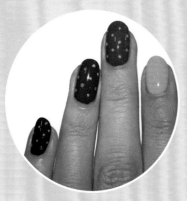

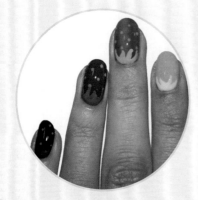

NAILS THAT LOOK GOOD ENOUGH TO EAT!

3 Once the base colours and polka dots have dried completely, you can add the strawberry leaves. Use four shades of green (from light to dark) to tone with the pink to red base colours. Using a small nail art brush begin by creating a 'U' shape at the base of each nail. Paint long and skinny triangles to resemble leaves – you can vary both size and length for each nail if you like.

4 Once your nail design is dry, seal it with top coat. Now you have nails so juicy you might just be tempted to take a bite!

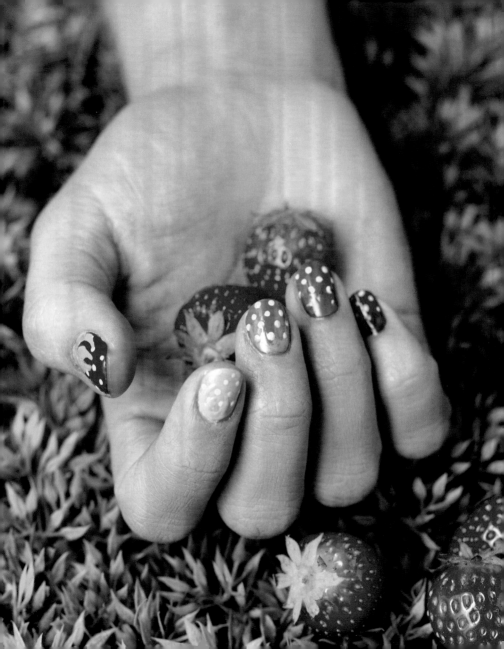

PINEAPPLE PARTY

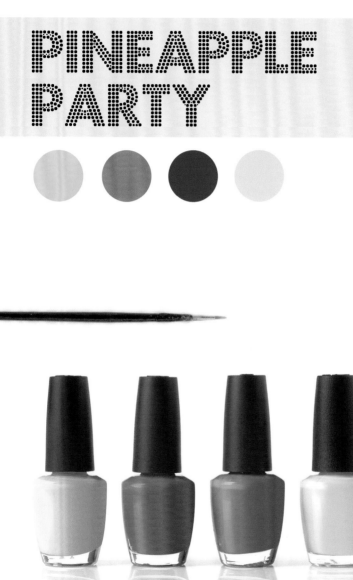

YOU WILL NEED

- Top and base coats
- Nail art brush shown

COLOURS

- Yellow
- Dark orange
- Dark green
- Light green

These tropical talons just scream **SUMMER**! This is a fairly advanced nail art design and might take a little bit more time than others but it's well worth it! Why not reward all your hard work with a suitably kitsch cocktail?

1 Apply a base coat and when dry, paint your nails with two coats of the yellow polish using the brush from the bottle.

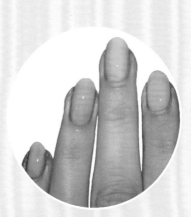

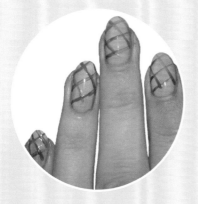

2 Using the nail art brush, use the orange polish to paint diagonal stripes from left to right and then cross over them to create a lattice pattern as shown. Stick with just a few strokes if you find it tricky at first, and add more as you get confident with the design. Allow to dry.

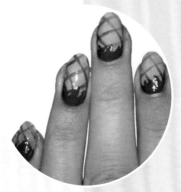

3 Take the dark green polish and, using the nail art brush, paint long and skinny triangles at the base of each nail. Make sure that they are uneven in length and shape as it will result in a better look.

4 Take the light green polish, and using a nail art brush, add highlights to the leaves with upward strokes from the base of the nail. Seal the nail design with a high-gloss top coat to finish. Ask the bartender to fix you a Mai Tai and relax – you're on vacation!

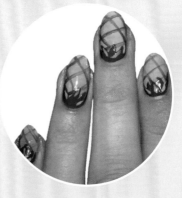

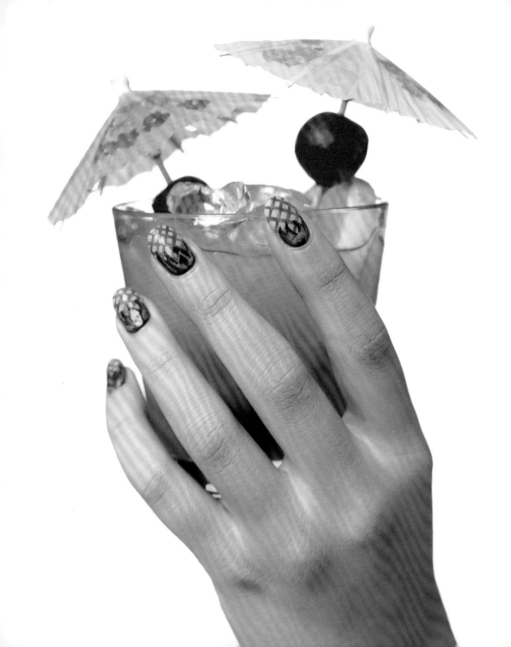

CRAZY CAT WOMAN

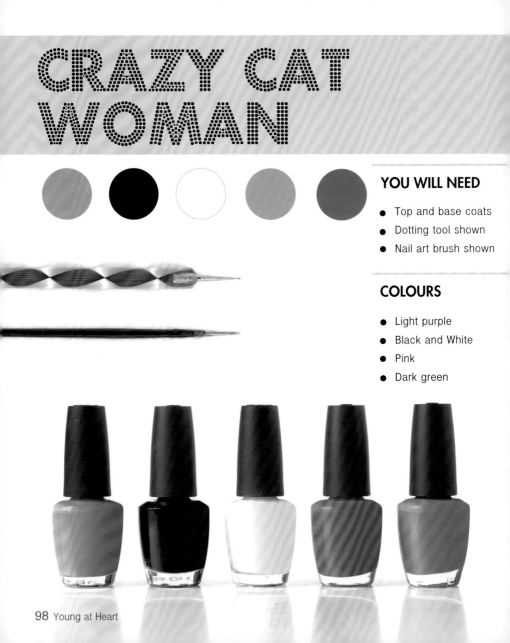

YOU WILL NEED

- Top and base coats
- Dotting tool shown
- Nail art brush shown

COLOURS

- Light purple
- Black and White
- Pink
- Dark green

Want to be **CUTER** than a basket of kittens? Here's how. You can play with this design by trying different colours for the fur and eyes, or even painting your own special kitty!

1 Apply a base coat and once dry, paint your nails with two coats of the purple polish.

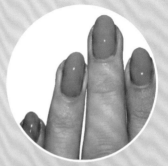

2 Take the black polish and using the brush from the bottle (or a nail art brush if preferred), begin creating the heads of the kittens by painting a semi-circle at the tip of each nail.

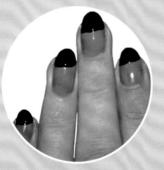

3 Once the shape of the head is complete, using a nail art brush, paint two tiny ears at the top of the semi-circle.

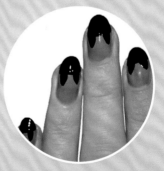

4 Using a nail art brush, paint two small ovals of white just under the ears of the cat to create the whites of the eyes.

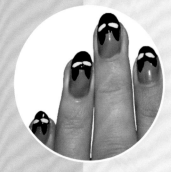

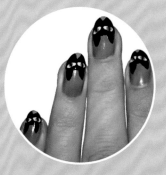

5 Add a dot of green to the white and when completely dry, add a last tiny dot of black to complete the eyes. Create little pink noses on all the kittens using a dotting tool.

6 Take the white polish and using a nail art brush, add two strokes either side of the nose to resemble whiskers and you're done! Once dry, seal with top coat. Now you are purrrrr-fect!

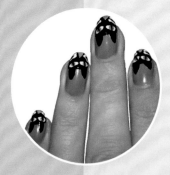

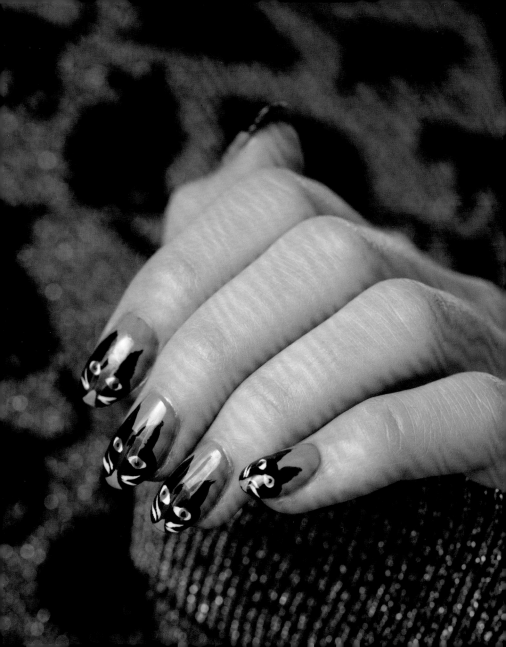

TUXEDO

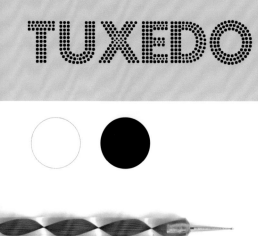

YOU WILL NEED

- Top and base coats
- Dotting tool shown
- Nail art brush shown

COLOURS

- White
- Black

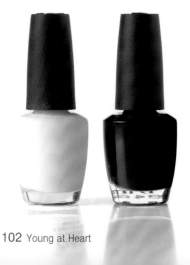

Before heading out the door to your next black-tie affair, make sure that your fingertips are as well-dressed as you are. This **TIMELESS** design is simple to achieve, yet ensures you will be truly dressed to impress whatever the event!

1 Apply a base coat and once dry, paint your nails all over with two coats of the white polish. Allow to dry completely.

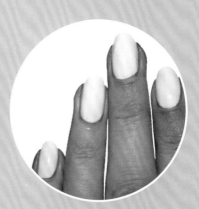

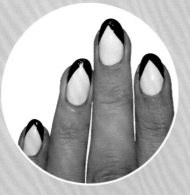

2 Take the black polish and, using a nail art brush and starting two-thirds of the way up one side of each nail, paint a thin diagonal line up to the centre tip. Repeat the process on the opposite side of the nail to create a 'V' shape. Using the brush from the polish bottle, fill in the triangle to create the jacket of the tuxedo.

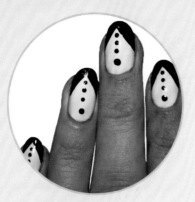

3 Using a dotting tool make three dots down the centre of the nail to create buttons. Take a very small nail art brush and create a figure eight shape at the base middle of each nail.

MAKE IT A BLACK-TIE AFFAIR!

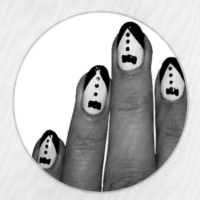

4 Carefully stretch out the figure eight, creating points at the edges to make a bow tie shape. Once the design has completely dried, apply a heavy-duty top coat. Now all you have to do is sit back and wait for your limo to arrive!

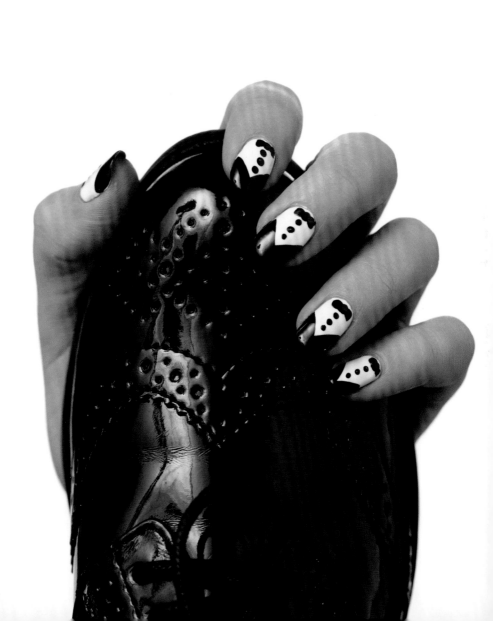

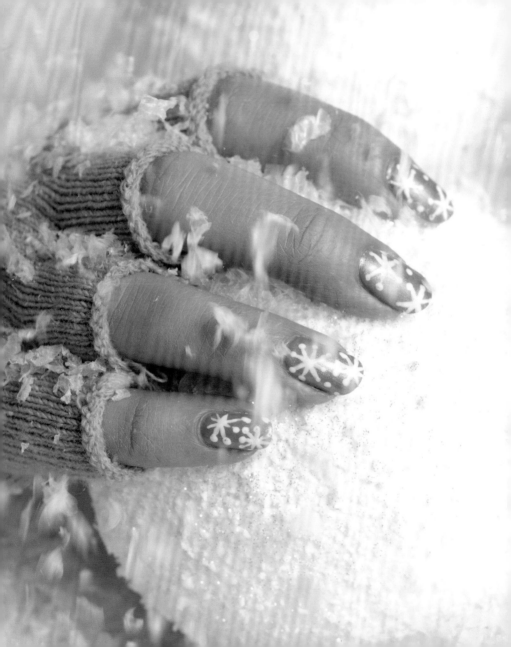

SEASONAL

SEASONAL

What better way to CELEBRATE the changing seasons than to decorate your nails with a nifty new design? Whether its Valentine's Day, Spring-time, Halloween or Christmas, here you'll find the perfect pattern to see you through each season in style.

I HEART YOU

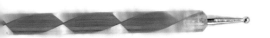

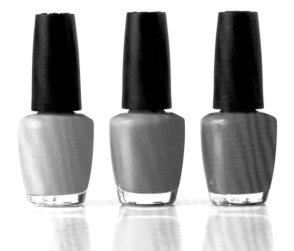

YOU WILL NEED

- Top and base coats
- Dotting tool shown

COLOURS

- Neutral
- Blue
- Purple

This is the perfect design for Valentine's Day, or any day that **LOVE** is in the air — why not try it for an anniversary? It's simple, and you can create plenty of looks by pairing different colours together for the hearts. Feel the love!

1 Apply a base coat and when dry, paint your nails with two coats of the neutral polish, using the brush from the polish bottle. Allow to dry.

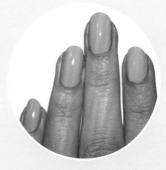

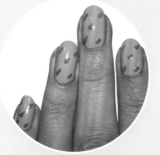

2 Take the purple polish and, using a small dotting tool make a dot anywhere on the nail and drag it down to a point — this will be the left-hand side of the heart shape. Repeat four times to create a scattered effect. (Do not worry about it looking perfect, as the blue polish on the right-hand side will cover up any mishaps.)

3 Take the blue polish and using a dotting tool, make a second dot beside each of the original ones and drag down to create a point. Once your nail design is dry, seal it with a high-shine top coat. Can you feel the love?

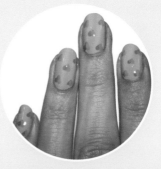

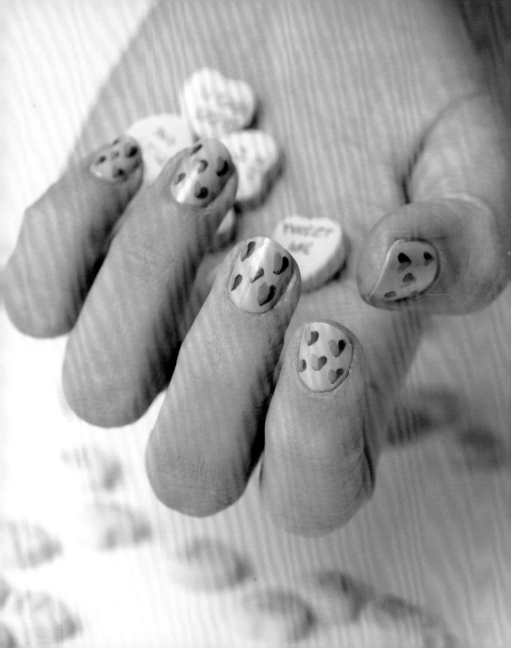

HIPPITY HOPPITY

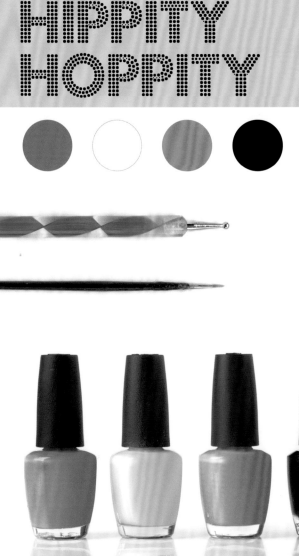

YOU WILL NEED

- Top and base coats
- Dotting tool shown
- Nail art brush shown

COLOURS

- Mauve
- White and black
- Pale pink

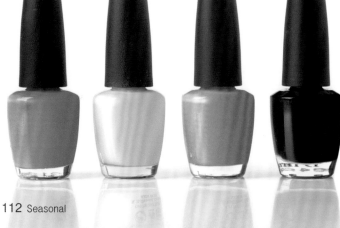

Are you ready for an **EASTER EGG** hunt? Give the Easter Bunny a run for his money with this super-cute design. If you find the technique a little tricky, you can always just create a solo bunny on an accent finger. Happy hunting!

1 Apply a base coat and when dry, paint each nail with two coats of the mauve polish, using the brush from the polish bottle.

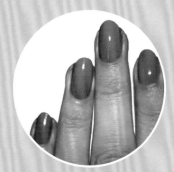

2 Take the white polish, and using the brush from the bottle, create a 'U' shape at the tip of each nail. You can use the bottle brush to create and fill in this shape.

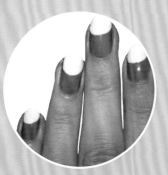

3 Using a thin nail art brush dipped in your white polish, create long, thin outlines for the ears of the bunny and fill them in.

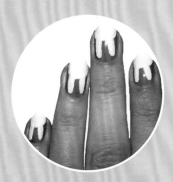

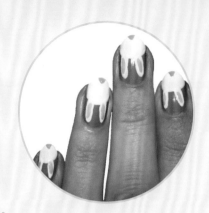

4 Clean off your nail art brush and dip it in the pale pink polish. Fill in the middle of the ears, still leaving a white outline around the edges and create a triangle shape for the nose at the tip of each nail.

THE HUNT IS ON!

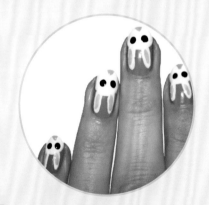

5 Using a dotting tool dipped in black polish, dot on the eyes. Seal with a heavy duty top coat, grab your egg hunt basket and join the search!

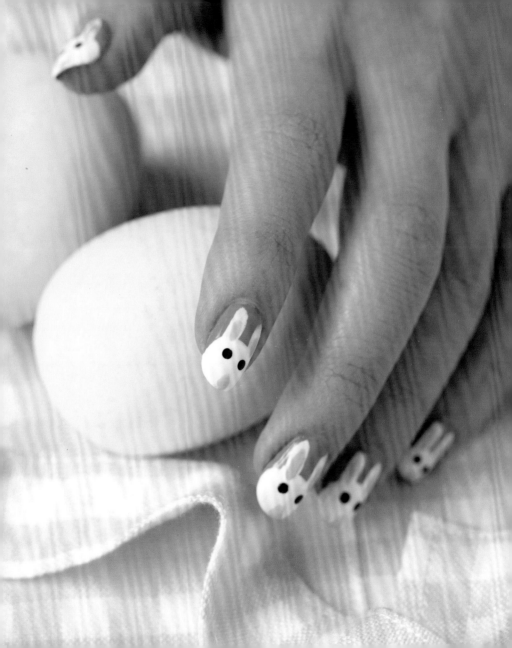

FRANKEN STITCHES

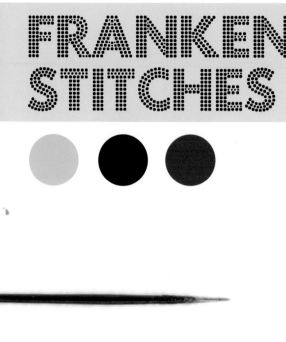

YOU WILL NEED

- Top and base coats
- Nail art brush shown

COLOURS

- Pale green
- Black
- Red

Learn a new **TRICK** and give your nails a **TREAT** this Halloween with this gruesome Frankenstein-inspired nail design. Easier to put together than a costume and still sure to scare every ghost and ghoul who crosses your path!

1 Apply a base coat and when dry, paint your nails with two coats of the pale green polish.

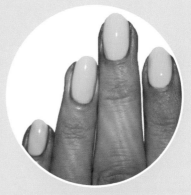

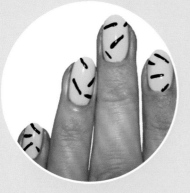

2 Take the black polish and, using a nail art brush, draw random, short lines at opposing angles across each nail.

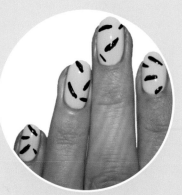

3 Add some Halloween gore by repeating this step with the red polish. Layering these colours makes these dashes look more like gashes!

4 Still using your nail art brush and black polish, paint shorter horizontal lines over the gashes to form stiches. Different lengths of stiches help perfect this look and create a handsewn look. What will it be this Halloween? Trick or treat – you choose...

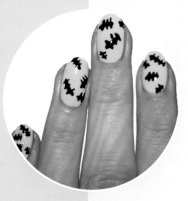

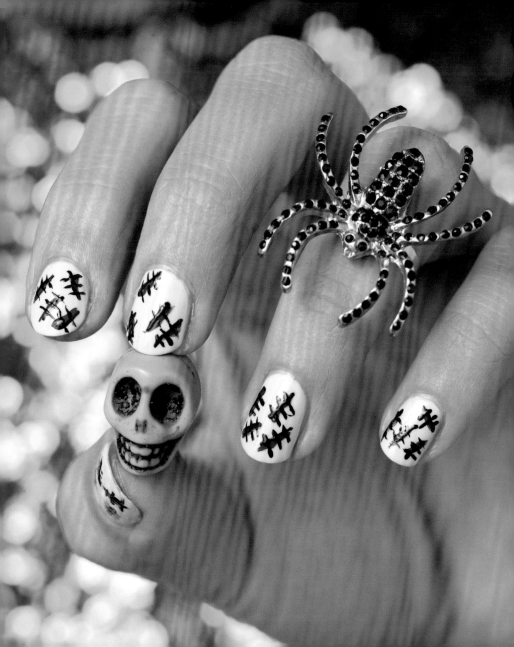

SNOWFLAKES

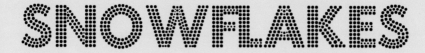

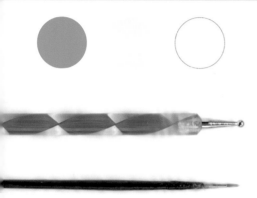

YOU WILL NEED

- Top and base coats
- Dotting tool shown
- Nail art brush shown

COLOURS

- Bright blue
- Shimmering blue
- Opaque white

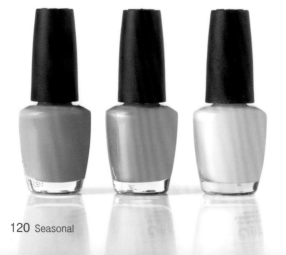

Baby it's **COLD** outside! Make every day a snow day with this cool-as-ice design. Don't forget to find your fingerless mittens though – you won't want to hide these fabulous frosty flakes away!

1 Apply a base coat and when dry, paint your nails with one coat of the bright blue polish and one coat of the metallic blue. Allow to dry completely.

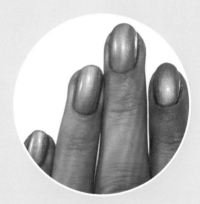

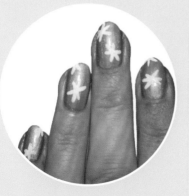

2 Take the white polish and, using a skinny nail art brush, paint three intersecting lines to create snowflakes. It works best to create a wide 'X' and then paint the third line across the middle. (Make sure not to place the lines too close together as it will make the next step more difficult.)

LET IT SNOW, LET IT SNOW, LET IT SNOW!

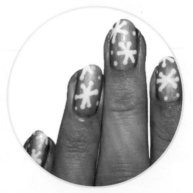

3 Using a dotting tool dipped in the white polish, add dots to the tips of each snowflake. Add a few random white dots across the nail for a full snowfall effect. Once the design is completely dry, go over the nail with a high-shine top coat or even a translucent glitter polish if you want to add some extra bling!

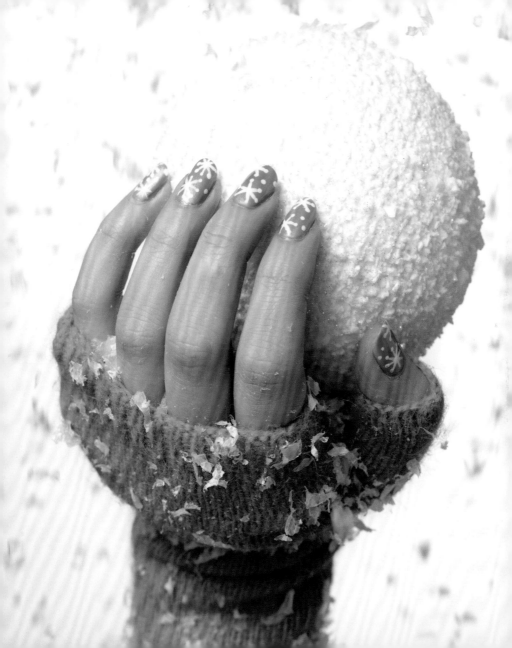

RESOURCES & SUPPLIERS

UK

WAH NAILS
420 Kingsland Road
London
E8 4AA
Visit www.wah-nails.com
London's original hipster nail bar where you can have whatever you want painted on your fingertips.

TOPSHOP
Visit www.topshop.com
One of Britain's best-loved fashion and beauty brands with stores all over the UK. With their very own line of nail art products Nails Topshop, including polishes, wraps, nail art pens and other useful tools, as well as their very own WAH Nail bar in London's flagship store.

NAILS INC.
Visit www.nailsinc.com
Award-winning fashion forward nail polish, nails care and services with nail bars and products in a variety of stores throughout the UK.

BEAUTY BAY
Visit
www.beautybay.com/nailcare
This online beauty store is a treasure trove of nail art products and polishes in a wide range of brands and colours.

SELFRIDGES
Visit www.selfridges.com
London's leading fashion and beauty department store stocking a wide range of nail products in a variety of the very best brands.

US

VALLEY
Visit www.valleynyc.com
Fashionable nail bar in Nolita, New York offering impeccable nail care, tips, gels and polish trends including hand-painted, 3-D acrylic and crystal designs.

PRIMP AND POLISH
Visit www.primpandpolish.com
Award-winning nail bar in New York's trendy Williamsburg offering a range of services including maincure, pedicures, gel manicures and nail art.

CHI NAIL BAR AND ORGANIC SPA
Visit www.chi-nailbar.com
One of LA's go-to nail bars for the stars, providing manicures, pedicures, nail art and a range of cutting-edge beauty treatments and techniques.

SPIFSTER NAILS
Visit
www.styleseat.com/spifstersutton
Spifster Sutton is a nail-design rock star based in Chicago, patiently painting outrageous, hipster-approved nail art in wild patterns and glittery Lady Gaga-style textures.

SEPHORA

Visit www.sephora.com
Sephora's beauty superstores throughout the US and Canada stock the most comprehensive range of beauty products including many brands of polishes and nail art tools.

CANADA

TRADE SECRETS CANADA

Visit www.tradesecrets.ca
for your nearest store.
Retailer of salon-quality hair, skin and beauty products. Offering over 4500 products and a full service salon, it's a one-stop beauty shop.

TIPS NAIL BAR

844a Danforth Avenue
Toronto, ON M4J 1L7
Visit www.tipsnailbar.ca
Experts in nail care. Tips Nail Bar offers technical expertise, boundless creativity and in demand services when it comes to nail care.

HOLT RENFREW

Visit www.holtrenfrew.com
for your nearest store.
Canadian department store selling a huge range of fashion and beauty products. Stocks a large selection of nail colours.

THE BAY

Visit www.thebay.com
for your nearest store.
Large department store in Canada offering a wide selection of the top names in fashion, beauty and home brands. Stocks a large selection of nail colours and brands.

BRANDS:

OPI

www.opi.com
Manufacturers of nail products for salon professionals. The professional OPI Nail Lacquer formula is available in over 200 fashion-forward colours.

ESSIE

www.essie.com
American brand specializing in high quality nail polish in a variety of fashionable colours. In addition to nail colour, Essie manufactures a full range of nail care products.

CHINA GLAZE

www.chinaglaze.com
Provider of globally rich, on-trend, innovative colour nail lacquers and treatments.

BOURJOIS

www.bourjois.co.uk
Parisian beauty brand specializing in feminine products that simplify beauty. Products include on-trend nail enamel and nail care products.

SALLY HANSEN

www.sallyhansen.com
Nail care mega brand specializing in nail treatment and colour. Provide innovative products that incorporate the latest treatment technologies.

INSPIRING BLOGS

polishyoupretty.com

Primacreative.com

Chalkboardnails.com

Heynicenails.com

Theillustratednail.tumblr.com

Wah-nails.com

Pshiiit.com

Missladyfinger.com

Polishartaddiction.blogspot.com

Freakynails.tumblr.com

Fashionpolish.com

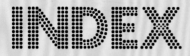

INDEX

AB
aloha 54–7
brushes 16

C
crazy cat woman 98–101

D
dotting
  polka dot power 24–7
  tools 12

F
floral designs 44–61
  aloha 54
  pretty peonies 58
  rosebuds 50
  smell the roses 47
franken stitches 116–18

HI
half moon 32–5
hippity hoppity 112–14
I heart you 109–10
ikat 72–4

L
leapin' leopard 68–71

MN
magic mixing 40–3
melting 87–8
nail art brushes 16

OP
ombre 21–3
pineapple party 94–6
polishes 10–11
polka dot power 24–7
pretty peonies 58–61
print designs 62–83
  ikat 72
  leopin' leopard 68
  tiger bright 65
  totally 80s 76
  tribal 80

R
resources and suppliers 124
rosebuds 50–54

S
sticky tape 14
seasonal designs 106–123
  franken stitches 116
  hippity hoppity 112
  I heart you 109
  snowflakes 120

simple designs 18–43
  half moon 32–5
  ombre 21–3
  magic mixing 40–3
  polka dot power 24–7
  splatter 28
  stained glass 36
smell the roses 47–50
snowflakes 120–3
splatter 28–31
sponges 14
stained glass 36–9
strawberry fields 90–3

T
tape, sticky 14
tiger bright 65–8
tools & techniques 6
totally 80s 76–9
tribal 80–2
tuxedo 102–5

Y
young at heart designs 84–105
  crazy cat woman 98
  melting 87
  pineapple party 94
  strawberry fields 90
  tuxedo 102

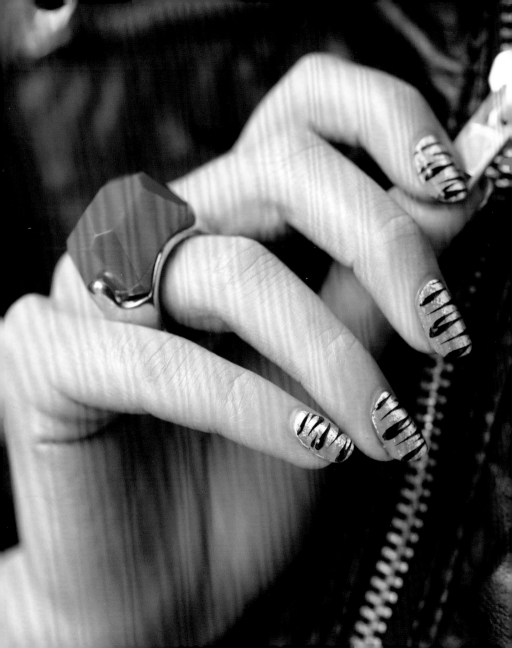

ACKNOWLEDGEMENTS

Who knew that this nail polish blog would turn into something so great? We are both so thankful to be able to put all of our hard work and passion into a project like this. We started our blog Polish You Pretty as our Creative outlet and to give us something productive to do with our growing nail polish collections, never imagining that it would be such a success. We'd like to thank all of our readers and supporters – our followers that spent time commenting on our post and e-mailing us with their feedback, and all the PR companies that sent us sample polish to keep our tutorials going. Without you we wouldn't be able to share our passion for nail art, so thank you.

A big thank you goes out to our friends who shared our posts with others and spread the word about Polish You Pretty – you are all absolutely amazing! We'd like to thank our parents; Donna and Peter, Nancy and Ed for pretending to understand what a blog was and even more so for pretending to understand why we would want write an entire blog about nail polish – you are our biggest fans! To our wonderful sisters Ashley and Emily who always did a good job at taking extra nail polish bottles off our hands, love you both. Thank you to our boyfriends – Shane and Scott, for putting up with the smell of nail polish almost every night, and pretending to understand the world of nail polish.

Last but not least, thank you to our nail polish sponsor, O.P.I. You've provided the world of nail polish with so many amazing shades and have been responsible for shaping polish trends in the past few years. Thank you for providing us with all the polish to complete these nail art designs – we couldn't of asked for a better sponsor!

We hope you all enjoy reading this book as much as we did writing it – keep polishing pretty.

Danielle & Jenny xo

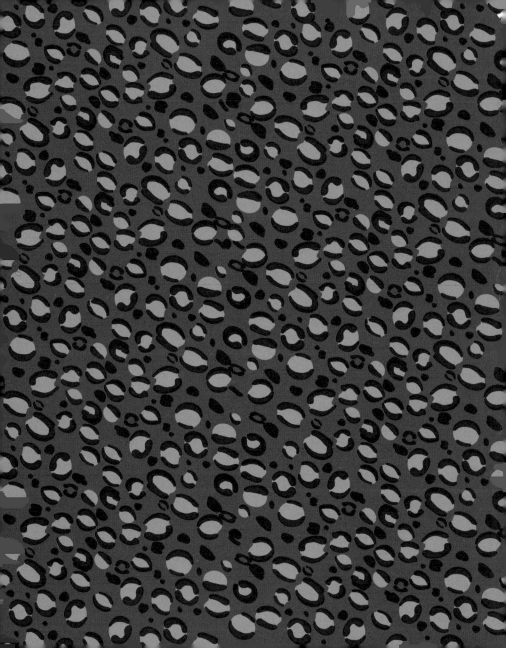